BDSM Sex Handbook

An Expert Guide to BDSM Sex for Beginners, Practical Tips from Sex Therapists and How BDSM Can Help Save Your Relationship

Cheryl Bach

BDSM Sex Handbook

Publisher: IntimateInk Press

Email: intimateinkpress@gmail.com

This book is a work of nonfiction intended for informational purposes only. The content of this book is based on the author's research, knowledge, and experience, and it is provided with the understanding that the author and publisher are not engaged in rendering legal, medical, or professional advice. The information in this book is not a substitute for professional guidance or assistance. Readers should consult with relevant professionals for advice and assistance regarding their specific situations. The author and publisher disclaim any liability for any loss or risk, personal or otherwise, which is incurred as a consequence, directly or indirectly, of the use and application of any of the contents of this book.

Cover design by IntimateInk Press

Interior layout and design by IntimateInk Press

Printed in USA

Fonts: Google fonts

Image: Freepik.com. This cover has been designed using assets from Freepik.com

For permission to use copyrighted material from this book, please contact the copyright holder listed above.

First Edition: 2024

Distributed by Amazon.com, Inc.

Cheryl Bach

Table of Contents

Cheryl Bach

Cheryl Bach

Chapter 1

Introduction

BDSM, an acronym that stands for Bondage, Discipline, Dominance, Submission, Sadism, and Masochism, is often a subject veiled in mystery, misconception, and even taboo. For many, the mere mention of BDSM conjures images of extreme practices portrayed in movies or exaggerated in media, leading to misunderstandings and fear. However, at its core, BDSM is a consensual and diverse spectrum of erotic practices that encompass a wide range of activities and dynamics.

In this introductory chapter, we embark on a journey to demystify BDSM, explore its significance in relationships, and lay the groundwork for understanding its principles and practices. We will delve into the importance of communication and consent within BDSM dynamics and provide an overview of what to expect in the subsequent chapters of this handbook.

Explanation of BDSM

BDSM is a multifaceted concept that encompasses various erotic activities and power dynamics. At its essence, BDSM involves consensual exploration of sexual desires and fantasies through the exchange of power, control, and sensation. It is not limited to physical acts but extends to psychological and emotional experiences as well.

Bondage: Bondage involves restraining a partner using ropes, restraints, or other tools to restrict movement. It can evoke feelings of vulnerability, trust, and excitement.

Discipline: Discipline in BDSM refers to the consensual use of punishment or rewards to modify behavior. It may involve activities such as spanking, paddling, or other forms of impact play.

Dominance and Submission: Dominance involves exerting control over a submissive partner, while submission entails willingly surrendering control. These roles are negotiated and may involve rituals, protocols, and obedience.

Sadism and Masochism: Sadism involves deriving pleasure from inflicting pain or humiliation on a consenting partner, whereas masochism involves deriving pleasure from receiving pain or humiliation. These activities are conducted with careful consideration for safety and boundaries.

Importance of Communication and Consent

Central to BDSM dynamics is the emphasis on communication and consent. Unlike the common misconception of BDSM as inherently abusive or non-consensual, practitioners of BDSM prioritize clear and ongoing communication to ensure that all parties involved are fully informed and consenting to the activities.

Communication: Effective communication involves expressing desires, limits, boundaries, and expectations openly and honestly with all partners involved. It allows individuals to negotiate scenes, establish protocols, and address any concerns or uncertainties.

Consent: Consent is the cornerstone of BDSM play and relationships. It must be informed, enthusiastic, and ongoing throughout all interactions. Consent can be given or revoked at any time, and respecting boundaries is paramount.

Cheryl Bach

Overview of the Book

In this comprehensive handbook, we aim to provide beginners with practical guidance and expert insights into navigating the world of BDSM. Drawing on the expertise of sex therapists, we offer practical tips, strategies, and exercises to help individuals explore their desires, enhance communication skills, and cultivate fulfilling BDSM experiences.

Each chapter of this book is designed to address specific aspects of BDSM, from understanding its fundamentals and exploring desires to building trust, practicing safety, and integrating BDSM into relationships. Whether you are curious about BDSM, seeking to enhance your sexual experiences, or looking to save your relationship through BDSM exploration, this handbook offers a wealth of knowledge and resources to support you on your journey.

As we embark on this exploration together, let us embrace curiosity, open-mindedness, and a commitment to mutual respect and consent. By understanding the principles of BDSM and cultivating healthy communication and consent practices, we can create safe, fulfilling, and transformative experiences that enrich our relationships and enhance our well-being.

Welcome to the BDSM Sex Handbook—a guide to unlocking the pleasures and possibilities of BDSM.

Chapter 2

Understanding BDSM

BDSM, often depicted in movies and books in sensationalized or inaccurate ways, is actually a diverse and complex world of human sexuality. In this chapter, we will explore the fundamental aspects of BDSM, its historical roots, dispel common myths, and delve into its profound psychological and emotional dimensions.

Defining BDSM

At its core, BDSM stands for Bondage, Discipline, Dominance, Submission, Sadism, and Masochism. Let's break down each element:

Bondage: Bondage involves the consensual restriction of movement using various tools like ropes, cuffs, or restraints. It can evoke feelings of vulnerability, trust, and intimacy between partners.

Discipline: Discipline in BDSM refers to the consensual use of punishment or rewards to modify behavior. It might involve activities such as spanking, paddling, or other forms of impact play, all negotiated beforehand.

Dominance and Submission: Dominance involves one partner taking control over the other, directing their actions, and orchestrating scenes according to agreed-upon terms. Submission, on the other hand, entails willingly surrendering control and obeying the dominant partner's commands. These roles are negotiated and can involve rituals, protocols, and power dynamics that deepen trust and intimacy.

Cheryl Bach

Sadism and Masochism: Sadism is the enjoyment of inflicting pain, humiliation, or control on a consenting partner, while masochism is the enjoyment of receiving those sensations. These activities are conducted with careful consideration for safety, consent, and boundaries, and can deepen the connection between partners.

History and Evolution of BDSM

BDSM has a long and varied history, with traces of its practices found in ancient cultures and throughout different time periods. From religious rituals to erotic literature, BDSM has evolved alongside human civilization. In modern times, it experienced a resurgence with the rise of underground subcultures and the publication of influential works like "The Story of O" and "Venus in Furs."

Debunking Myths and Misconceptions

Despite its growing acceptance, BDSM is still surrounded by myths and misconceptions. One common myth is that it's abusive or non-consensual. In reality, BDSM is based on trust, communication, and mutual consent. It's not about causing harm but exploring desires in a safe and consensual manner.

Psychological and Emotional Aspects of BDSM

Beneath the surface of BDSM lies a rich landscape of psychological and emotional dynamics. Engaging in BDSM activities can provide a unique avenue for self-expression, self-discovery, and personal growth. It can help individuals explore aspects of themselves that may be taboo or suppressed in mainstream society.

Furthermore, the power dynamics inherent in BDSM can foster feelings of trust, vulnerability, and emotional intimacy between partners. Research suggests that engaging in BDSM activities can lead to increased self-esteem, stress relief, and improved mood.

In conclusion, understanding BDSM involves recognizing its diverse components, understanding its historical context, dispelling myths, and acknowledging its psychological and emotional dimensions. By embracing these aspects, individuals can embark on a journey of exploration and discovery that can enrich their relationships and enhance their well-being.

Chapter 3

Exploring Your Desires

Embarking on a journey into the world of BDSM can be both exhilarating and daunting. In this chapter, we'll guide you through the process of exploring your desires, understanding your sexual preferences, identifying your limits and boundaries, and learning how to negotiate and communicate effectively with your partners. By taking the time to reflect on your desires and communicate openly with your partners, you can embark on a journey of self-discovery and mutual exploration that is both fulfilling and empowering.

Self-Reflection and Understanding Your Sexual Preferences

Before diving into BDSM play, it's essential to take some time for self-reflection and introspection. Understanding your own desires, fantasies, and boundaries is crucial for navigating the diverse landscape of BDSM activities and dynamics.

Here are some steps you can take to explore your desires:

Reflect on past experiences: Think about any experiences you've had that made you feel excited, intrigued, or aroused. What aspects of those experiences appealed to you? What fantasies or desires have you never acted on but find intriguing?

Explore fantasies: Fantasies are a natural part of human sexuality and can provide valuable insights into your desires. Take some time to explore your fantasies, whether through daydreaming, journaling, or discussing them with a trusted partner.

Consider your boundaries: Think about what activities or experiences you feel comfortable exploring and what activities you prefer to avoid. Remember that boundaries can change over time and vary depending on the context and your partner(s).

Identify your preferences: Take note of any specific activities, roles, or dynamics that pique your interest. Are you drawn to the idea of being dominant, submissive, or switching between roles? Do you have preferences for particular sensations, such as pain, restraint, or sensory deprivation?

Identifying Limits and Boundaries

Setting clear limits and boundaries is essential for ensuring that BDSM play is safe, consensual, and enjoyable for all parties involved. Your limits are the things you absolutely do not want to do or experience, while boundaries are the lines you don't want to cross in terms of intensity or duration.

Here are some tips for identifying your limits and boundaries:

Consider physical and emotional boundaries: Think about what activities or sensations you are comfortable with physically and emotionally. Are there any specific acts or scenarios that trigger anxiety, discomfort, or trauma?

Communicate with yourself: Listen to your instincts and pay attention to your body's reactions. If something doesn't feel right or causes you distress, it's important to acknowledge and respect those feelings.

Be honest with yourself: Don't feel pressured to conform to expectations or engage in activities that don't align with your desires or comfort level. It's okay to say no to things that don't feel right for you.

Discuss boundaries with your partner(s): Once you've identified your own limits and boundaries, communicate them openly and honestly with your partner(s). Encourage them to do the same so that you can establish mutual trust and respect.

Negotiation and Communication with Partners

Effective communication is the cornerstone of healthy BDSM dynamics. Negotiating scenes, setting boundaries, and discussing preferences with your partner(s) are essential for ensuring that everyone's needs and desires are respected.

Here are some strategies for negotiating and communicating effectively:

Initiate open dialogue: Start by expressing your interest in exploring BDSM and initiating an open dialogue with your partner(s) about their thoughts, feelings, and boundaries.

Use clear language: Be specific and clear when discussing your desires, limits, and boundaries. Use concrete examples and descriptive language to ensure mutual understanding.

Listen actively: Take the time to listen to your partner(s) without judgment or interruption. Validate their feelings and concerns and demonstrate empathy and understanding.

Seek consent: Consent is essential in BDSM play and should be given freely, enthusiastically, and continuously. Check in with your partner(s) regularly during play to ensure that everyone is comfortable and consenting.

By taking the time to explore your desires, communicate openly with your partner(s), and establish clear boundaries, you can embark on a journey of mutual exploration and discovery that is both fulfilling and empowering. Remember that BDSM is a journey, and it's okay to take things slow, ask questions, and seek support along the way.

Chapter 4

Building Trust and Consent

Trust and consent are the cornerstones of healthy and fulfilling BDSM dynamics. In this chapter, we will explore the importance of trust in BDSM relationships, the various ways to establish and maintain consent, and the crucial role of safe words and signals in ensuring safety and communication.

Importance of Trust in BDSM Dynamics

Trust forms the foundation of any successful BDSM relationship. Without trust, it's impossible to fully surrender to the vulnerability and intensity of BDSM play. Building trust takes time and effort, but it's essential for creating a safe and secure environment where both partners can explore their desires freely.

Vulnerability: BDSM often involves exploring intense emotions, fantasies, and sensations. Trust allows individuals to be vulnerable with their partners, knowing that they will be supported and respected.

Communication: Trust encourages open and honest communication between partners. It enables individuals to express their desires, boundaries, and concerns without fear of judgment or rejection.

Safety: Trust ensures that both partners feel safe and cared for during BDSM play. It allows individuals to push their boundaries and explore new experiences knowing that their partner has their best interests at heart.

Establishing Consent: Verbal, Non-Verbal, and Continuous

Consent is the cornerstone of ethical BDSM play. It's not just about saying "yes" to a particular activity—it's about ongoing communication and mutual agreement.

Here are some key aspects of establishing consent in BDSM:

Verbal Consent: Verbal communication is the most direct way to establish consent. Before engaging in any BDSM activity, partners should clearly communicate their desires, limits, and boundaries. This can involve discussing specific activities, using descriptive language, and asking for explicit permission.

Non-Verbal Cues: In addition to verbal consent, partners should pay attention to non-verbal cues such as body language, facial expressions, and vocalizations. These cues can provide valuable insights into how someone is feeling and whether they are comfortable with the current activity.

Continuous Consent: Consent is not a one-time event—it's an ongoing process that requires constant communication and awareness. Throughout BDSM play, partners should check in with each other regularly to ensure that everyone is still comfortable and consenting. This can involve asking questions, using reassuring gestures, or using predetermined signals.

Safe Words and Safe Signals

Safe words and signals are essential tools for communicating boundaries and ensuring safety during BDSM play. They provide a way for individuals to indicate when they want to stop or pause an activity, even if they are unable to speak.

Here's how they work:

Choosing a Safe Word: A safe word is a word or phrase that is used to indicate when someone wants to stop or pause a BDSM activity. It should be something that is easy to remember and unlikely to be confused with normal conversation. Common safe words include "red" for stop and "yellow" for slow down or check-in.

Using Safe Signals: In addition to safe words, partners can also use safe signals to communicate non-verbally. This can involve using hand gestures, tapping out a rhythm, or dropping a specific object as a signal to stop.

Respecting Safe Words and Signals: It's essential for partners to respect safe words and signals without question. If someone uses a safe word or signal, it means that they are no longer comfortable with the activity, and it should be stopped immediately.

By prioritizing trust and consent, and using safe words and signals effectively, individuals can create a safe and empowering environment for exploring BDSM play. In the next chapter, we'll delve deeper into practical BDSM techniques and activities, with a focus on safety and communication.

Chapter 5

BDSM Practices and Techniques

BDSM encompasses a wide array of practices and techniques that cater to diverse desires and fantasies. In this chapter, we will explore some of the most common BDSM activities, including bondage, discipline, dominance and submission, sadism and masochism, and sensation play. Whether you're a curious beginner or an experienced practitioner, understanding these practices and techniques can enhance your BDSM experiences and deepen your connection with your partner(s).

Bondage: Rope, Restraints, and Shibari

Bondage is a popular BDSM activity that involves the consensual restraint of a partner using various tools and techniques.

Here are some key aspects of bondage:

Rope Bondage: Rope bondage, also known as shibari or kinbaku, involves using ropes to create intricate patterns and designs on the body. It requires skill and practice to tie safely and effectively, but it can be incredibly rewarding for both the rigger (person tying) and the bottom (person being tied).

Restraints: Restraints come in many forms, including cuffs, chains, straps, and bondage tape. They are used to restrict movement and create a sense of vulnerability and helplessness in the submissive partner.

Shibari: Shibari is a Japanese style of rope bondage that focuses on aesthetics, precision, and emotional connection.

It emphasizes the beauty of the ties and the intimacy between the rigger and the bottom.

Discipline: Spanking, Paddling, and Impact Play

Discipline in BDSM involves the consensual use of punishment or rewards to modify behavior and enhance erotic experiences.

Here are some common forms of discipline:

Spanking: Spanking is one of the most basic and popular forms of impact play. It involves striking the buttocks or other parts of the body with an open hand or a paddle. Spanking can range from gentle and sensual to intense and stingy, depending on the preferences of the participants.

Paddling: Paddling involves using a paddle or similar implement to strike the body. Paddles come in various shapes, sizes, and materials, each producing different sensations. Paddling can be administered as part of a scene or as a form of punishment in a disciplinary context.

Impact Play: Impact play includes a wide range of activities involving striking the body with various implements, such as floggers, canes, whips, and crops. It can be sensual, cathartic, or intense, depending on the preferences and limits of the participants.

Dominance and Submission: Power Dynamics and Role-Playing

Dominance and submission are central themes in BDSM dynamics, involving power exchange and role-playing.

Here's what you need to know:

Power Dynamics: Power dynamics refer to the consensual exchange of control between partners. Dominants (or tops) take on the role of authority figures, directing scenes and making decisions, while submissives (or bottoms) relinquish control and follow their partner's lead.

Role-Playing: Role-playing involves adopting specific roles or personas within a BDSM scene. This can include scenarios such as teacher/student, boss/employee, or master/slave, among others. Role-playing allows participants to explore different dynamics and fantasies in a safe and consensual way.

Sadism and Masochism: Understanding Pain Play

Sadism and masochism involve deriving pleasure from giving or receiving pain, respectively.

Here's how they play out in BDSM:

Sadism: Sadists enjoy inflicting pain, humiliation, or control on a consenting partner. This can involve activities such as spanking, biting, scratching, or using implements like whips or paddles. Sadistic play should always be negotiated and conducted with care and respect for the masochist's limits.

Masochism: Masochists derive pleasure from receiving pain, humiliation, or control. They may enjoy sensations ranging from mild discomfort to intense pain, depending on their preferences. Masochistic play should always be negotiated and conducted with care and attention to the masochist's safety and well-being.

Sensation Play: Temperature, Sensory Deprivation, and Wax Play

Sensation play involves exploring different sensations and stimuli to enhance erotic experiences.

Here are some common forms of sensation play:

Temperature Play: Temperature play involves using hot or cold objects, substances, or environments to stimulate the body. This can include ice cubes, hot wax, cold metal, or temperature-controlled toys. Temperature play can create intense sensations and enhance arousal.

Sensory Deprivation: Sensory deprivation involves limiting or removing one or more senses to heighten awareness and sensitivity. This can include blindfolding, gagging, earplugs, or sensory deprivation hoods. Sensory deprivation can intensify other sensations and create a sense of vulnerability and anticipation.

Wax Play: Wax play involves dripping hot wax onto the body and then removing it or playing with it. It can create a range of sensations, from gentle warmth to intense heat, depending on the type of wax used and the height from which it's dripped. Wax play requires caution and communication to ensure safety and enjoyment.

Understanding these BDSM practices and techniques can help you explore your desires, communicate effectively with your partner(s), and enhance your BDSM experiences. Remember to prioritize safety, communication, and consent at all times, and always respect your partner's limits and boundaries. In the following chapters, we'll delve deeper into practical tips and strategies for engaging in BDSM play safely and responsibly.

Chapter 6

Safety and Risk Management

Engaging in BDSM play can be exciting and fulfilling, but it's essential to prioritize safety and risk management to ensure a positive and enjoyable experience for all involved. In this chapter, we will explore various aspects of safety, including physical safety, emotional safety, and safer sex practices, to help you navigate BDSM play safely and responsibly.

Physical Safety: Injury Prevention and First Aid

Communication and Consent: Open and honest communication between partners is crucial for ensuring physical safety during BDSM play. Before engaging in any activities, discuss boundaries, limits, and preferences to avoid misunderstandings or accidents.

Education and Training: If you're new to BDSM or trying out new techniques, educate yourself about safety guidelines and best practices. Consider attending workshops, reading books, or seeking guidance from experienced practitioners to learn proper techniques and risk management strategies.

Risk Awareness: Be aware of the potential risks associated with different BDSM activities, such as impact play, bondage, and sensation play. Take steps to minimize risks, such as using safe words, checking for signs of distress, and using appropriate safety equipment.

Injury Prevention: Take precautions to prevent injuries during BDSM play, such as using padded surfaces for impact play, avoiding joints and sensitive areas when striking, and maintaining proper body mechanics when engaging in physical activities.

First Aid: Have a basic understanding of first aid principles and know how to respond to common injuries that may occur during BDSM play, such as bruises, abrasions, or rope burns. Keep a first aid kit handy and seek medical attention if needed.

Emotional Safety: Aftercare and Debriefing

Aftercare: Aftercare is a crucial aspect of emotional safety in BDSM play. It involves providing emotional support, comfort, and reassurance to both partners after a scene to help them transition back to a state of emotional equilibrium. Aftercare can include physical affection, cuddling, verbal affirmations, and check-ins.

Debriefing: Debriefing allows partners to discuss their thoughts, feelings, and experiences after a scene in a safe and supportive environment. It provides an opportunity to process emotions, address any concerns or issues that may have arisen during play, and reinforce feelings of trust and connection.

Check-Ins: Check-ins are ongoing conversations that occur before, during, and after BDSM play to ensure that everyone feels safe, comfortable, and respected. Check in with your partner(s) regularly to gauge their emotional state and address any concerns or boundaries that may arise.

Safer Sex Practices in BDSM

Barrier Methods: When engaging in activities that involve bodily fluids or mucous membranes, such as oral sex, penetration, or fluid exchange, use barrier methods such as condoms, dental dams, or gloves to reduce the risk of sexually transmitted infections (STIs) and other communicable diseases.

Hygiene Practices: Maintain good hygiene practices before and after BDSM play, such as washing your hands, cleaning toys and equipment, and practicing safe body hygiene. Avoid sharing toys or equipment without proper cleaning and disinfection.

Regular Testing: Get tested for STIs regularly, especially if you engage in BDSM play with multiple partners or participate in high-risk activities. Encourage your partners to do the same and have open discussions about sexual health and testing.

Negotiation and Disclosure: When entering into BDSM play with a new partner, disclose any relevant medical history, STI status, or other health concerns. Discuss safer sex practices, boundaries, and expectations beforehand to ensure mutual understanding and consent.

By prioritizing physical safety, emotional well-being, and safer sex practices, you can enjoy BDSM play with confidence, knowing that you're taking proactive steps to mitigate risks and protect yourself and your partner(s). Remember that safety is an ongoing process that requires communication, awareness, and mutual respect. In the next chapter, we'll delve deeper into practical tips and strategies for enhancing safety and risk management in BDSM play.

Chapter 7

BDSM and Relationships

BDSM can add depth, excitement, and intimacy to relationships, whether they're long-standing or newly formed. In this chapter, we'll explore how to incorporate BDSM into existing relationships, navigate BDSM dynamics in new relationships, and communicate effectively to resolve conflicts and strengthen your bond.

Incorporating BDSM into Existing Relationships

Open Communication: The key to successfully incorporating BDSM into an existing relationship is open communication. Start by discussing your desires, fantasies, and boundaries with your partner(s) in a non-judgmental and supportive environment. Share what intrigues you about BDSM and ask for your partner's thoughts and feelings.

Exploring Together: Take a collaborative approach to exploring BDSM by experimenting with different activities and dynamics together. Start slowly and gradually introduce new elements as you both feel comfortable. Remember to prioritize each other's pleasure, safety, and emotional well-being throughout the process.

Negotiation and Consent: Negotiate scenes and activities with your partner(s) to ensure that everyone's desires, limits, and boundaries are respected. Use safe words and signals to communicate during play and check in with each other regularly to gauge comfort levels and make adjustments as needed.

Aftercare and Debriefing: Incorporate aftercare and debriefing into your BDSM play to provide emotional support and reassurance to each other after a scene. Use this time to cuddle, talk, and reconnect on an emotional level, reinforcing feelings of trust and intimacy.

Exploring BDSM Dynamics in New Relationships

Building Trust: Trust is essential in any relationship but especially important when exploring BDSM dynamics. Take the time to build trust with your new partner(s) through open communication, honesty, and reliability. Start slowly and gradually explore BDSM activities together as you get to know each other better.

Negotiating Boundaries: Negotiate boundaries and limits with your new partner(s) before engaging in BDSM play. Discuss each other's desires, fantasies, and comfort levels to ensure that everyone feels safe and respected. Be willing to compromise and adjust your expectations as needed.

Establishing Roles: Determine your roles and dynamics within the BDSM relationship, whether you identify as dominant, submissive, or switch. Be clear about your expectations and preferences and listen to your partner(s) to understand their desires and boundaries.

Navigating Power Dynamics: Power dynamics can be complex and nuanced in BDSM relationships. Take the time to explore power exchange dynamics with your partner(s) and establish protocols and rituals that enhance trust and intimacy. Remember to prioritize consent and mutual respect in all interactions.

Communication and Conflict Resolution in BDSM Relationships

Effective Communication: Communication is key to resolving conflicts and maintaining a healthy BDSM relationship. Practice active listening, empathy, and non-defensive communication techniques to express your needs and concerns openly and honestly. Be willing to listen to your partner(s) and validate their feelings and perspectives.

Conflict Resolution: When conflicts arise, address them promptly and constructively. Use "I" statements to express how you feel and avoid blaming or criticizing your partner(s). Collaborate on finding solutions that satisfy both of your needs and interests, and be willing to compromise when necessary.

Rebuilding Trust: If trust is breached in a BDSM relationship, take steps to rebuild it through transparency, accountability, and consistent communication. Be willing to acknowledge mistakes, apologize sincerely, and work together to repair the relationship.

Seeking Support: If you're struggling to navigate conflicts or communication challenges in your BDSM relationship, consider seeking support from a therapist or counselor who specializes in BDSM or alternative lifestyles. Professional guidance can provide valuable insights and strategies for overcoming obstacles and strengthening your relationship.

By incorporating BDSM into your relationship, whether existing or new, and prioritizing open communication, negotiation, and mutual respect, you can deepen your connection with your partner(s) and experience greater fulfillment and intimacy in your relationship. In the next chapter, we'll explore practical tips and techniques for enhancing pleasure and satisfaction in BDSM play.

Chapter 8

Overcoming Challenges

BDSM can be a source of pleasure, intimacy, and personal growth, but it's not without its challenges. In this chapter, we'll explore how to overcome common obstacles and navigate the complexities of societal judgments, jealousy, and relationship issues within BDSM dynamics.

Dealing with Societal Judgments and Stigma

Understanding Society's Views: Recognize that BDSM is still stigmatized in many societies due to misconceptions, stereotypes, and moral judgments. Understand that societal attitudes towards BDSM may influence your own perceptions and feelings about your desires and practices.

Educating Yourself and Others: Educate yourself about BDSM and its diverse practices, values, and communities. Challenge stereotypes and misinformation by engaging in open and respectful conversations with friends, family, and peers. Share accurate information and personal experiences to combat stigma and promote understanding.

Seeking Support: Surround yourself with supportive and accepting individuals who respect your choices and lifestyle. Seek out BDSM-friendly communities, forums, and events where you can connect with like-minded individuals and receive validation and encouragement.

Self-Validation: Validate your own desires and choices by embracing your sexuality and identity without shame or judgment. Remember that your worth and happiness are not determined by societal norms or expectations. Focus on cultivating self-acceptance, confidence, and empowerment in your BDSM journey.

Handling Jealousy and Insecurities

Understanding Jealousy: Jealousy is a natural emotion that can arise in any relationship, including BDSM dynamics. Understand that jealousy often stems from feelings of insecurity, fear of loss, or comparison with others. Acknowledge your feelings without judgment and explore their underlying causes.

Communicating Openly: Open communication is essential for addressing jealousy and insecurities in BDSM relationships. Share your feelings with your partner(s) in a non-blaming and non-defensive manner. Be honest about your fears and concerns and listen empathetically to your partner(s) without judgment.

Building Trust: Strengthen trust in your relationship by demonstrating reliability, honesty, and transparency. Keep your promises, respect your partner's boundaries, and communicate openly about your desires and intentions. Reassure your partner(s) of your commitment and loyalty through words and actions.

Self-Reflection and Self-Care: Take time to reflect on your own insecurities and triggers and practice self-care techniques to manage them effectively. Engage in activities that boost your self-esteem and confidence, such as hobbies, exercise, and mindfulness practices. Prioritize your emotional well-being and seek support from friends, therapists, or support groups if needed.

Addressing Common Relationship Issues in BDSM Dynamics

Power Imbalance: Recognize that power dynamics inherent in BDSM relationships can sometimes lead to imbalances or conflicts. Discuss power dynamics openly with your partner(s) and establish clear boundaries, protocols, and mechanisms for addressing power differentials.

Communication Breakdowns: Communication breakdowns can occur in any relationship, but they can be especially challenging in BDSM dynamics where trust and consent are paramount. Practice active listening, empathy, and assertive communication techniques to overcome communication barriers and resolve conflicts effectively.

Mismatched Expectations: Clarify expectations, desires, and boundaries with your partner(s) to ensure alignment and avoid misunderstandings or disappointments. Discuss your fantasies, preferences, and limits openly and negotiate mutually satisfying agreements that prioritize consent and respect.

Navigating Changes and Transitions: Recognize that BDSM dynamics, like any relationship, may evolve and change over time. Be flexible and adaptable in navigating transitions, life changes, or shifts in desires or boundaries. Communicate openly with your partner(s) about your needs, concerns, and aspirations and collaborate on finding solutions that accommodate both of your needs.

By confronting societal judgments, addressing jealousy and insecurities, and navigating common relationship challenges with honesty, empathy, and resilience, you can overcome obstacles and cultivate a fulfilling and sustainable BDSM relationship. In the next chapter, we'll explore practical strategies and techniques for enhancing intimacy, pleasure, and connection in BDSM play.

Chapter 9

BDSM and Mental Health

BDSM is not only a source of pleasure and intimacy but can also have therapeutic benefits for individuals seeking self-exploration, healing, and personal growth. In this chapter, we'll delve into the therapeutic benefits of BDSM, how it can be used as a tool for self-exploration and healing, and how to find BDSM-friendly therapists who can provide professional support.

Therapeutic Benefits of BDSM

Empowerment: Engaging in BDSM activities can empower individuals by allowing them to explore and embrace their desires, fantasies, and identities without judgment or shame. Taking ownership of one's sexuality and desires can foster self-confidence, self-esteem, and self-acceptance.

Stress Relief: BDSM play can provide a release valve for stress, tension, and anxiety by allowing individuals to escape from everyday worries and responsibilities and focus on the present moment. The intensity of BDSM activities can create a sense of catharsis and relaxation, leading to reduced stress levels and improved mood.

Emotional Release: BDSM play can offer an outlet for expressing and processing intense emotions, traumas, and psychological struggles in a safe and controlled environment. Activities like impact play, role-playing, and power exchange can help individuals explore and release pent-up emotions and experiences.

Connection and Intimacy: BDSM dynamics emphasize trust, communication, and vulnerability, fostering deep emotional connections and intimacy between partners. Engaging in BDSM activities can enhance emotional bonding, communication skills, and mutual understanding, leading to stronger and more fulfilling relationships.

Using BDSM as a Tool for Self-Exploration and Healing

Exploring Desires and Boundaries: BDSM provides a structured framework for exploring desires, fantasies, and boundaries in a consensual and safe manner. By engaging in BDSM activities, individuals can gain insights into their preferences, limits, and emotional responses, leading to greater self-awareness and self-discovery.

Processing Trauma: BDSM can be a therapeutic tool for processing past traumas, including abuse, neglect, or other adverse experiences. Through activities like role-playing, sensation play, and power exchange, individuals can reclaim agency, rewrite narratives, and heal emotional wounds in a supportive and empowering context.

Building Resilience: BDSM encourages individuals to confront fears, push boundaries, and challenge preconceived notions about themselves and their capabilities. By facing challenges and overcoming obstacles in BDSM play, individuals can build resilience, confidence, and coping skills that translate into other areas of their lives.

Embracing Authenticity: BDSM fosters authenticity and self-expression by encouraging individuals to embrace their true desires, identities, and vulnerabilities without judgment or inhibition. By embracing authenticity in BDSM play, individuals can cultivate a sense of wholeness, authenticity, and fulfillment in their lives.

Seeking Professional Help: Finding BDSM-Friendly Therapists

Research and Networking: Seek out therapists who specialize in sex therapy, kink-aware therapy, or alternative lifestyles. Research online directories, professional organizations, and community forums for therapists who are knowledgeable and accepting of BDSM practices.

Interviewing Therapists: When seeking therapy, interview potential therapists to ensure they are knowledgeable, non-judgmental, and supportive of BDSM lifestyles. Ask about their experience working with clients in BDSM relationships and their approach to addressing sexual and relationship issues.

Building Trust: Establish trust and rapport with your therapist by being open and honest about your BDSM practices, desires, and concerns. A BDSM-friendly therapist should create a safe and accepting space for discussing sensitive topics without shame or stigma.

Seeking Support Groups: Consider joining support groups, online forums, or community organizations for individuals in BDSM relationships. These groups can provide peer support, resources, and referrals to BDSM-friendly therapists who understand the unique challenges and dynamics of BDSM relationships.

By recognizing the therapeutic benefits of BDSM, using it as a tool for self-exploration and healing, and seeking support from BDSM-friendly therapists, individuals can cultivate greater self-awareness, resilience, and authenticity in their lives and relationships. In the next chapter, we'll explore practical techniques and strategies for enhancing pleasure, communication, and intimacy in BDSM play.

Chapter 10

Conclusion

In this comprehensive guide to BDSM sex, we've covered a wide range of topics, from understanding BDSM dynamics to navigating challenges and exploring the therapeutic benefits of BDSM. As we wrap up this handbook, let's recap the key points, offer encouragement for continued exploration and growth in BDSM, and reflect on the potential of BDSM to enhance relationships and personal well-being.

Recap of Key Points

Understanding BDSM: We explored the fundamental elements of BDSM, including bondage, discipline, dominance and submission, sadism and masochism, and sensation play. Understanding these aspects is essential for safe and fulfilling BDSM experiences.

Communication and Consent: We emphasized the importance of open communication, negotiation, and consent in BDSM dynamics. Clear communication and mutual agreement are essential for building trust, respecting boundaries, and ensuring safety.

Safety and Risk Management: We discussed strategies for maintaining physical safety, emotional well-being, and practicing safer sex in BDSM play. Prioritizing safety, risk awareness, and aftercare are essential for positive BDSM experiences.

Overcoming Challenges: We addressed common challenges in BDSM, such as societal judgments, jealousy, and relationship issues, and provided strategies for navigating them effectively. Open communication, trust-building, and self-reflection are key to overcoming obstacles in BDSM relationships.

BDSM and Mental Health: We explored the therapeutic benefits of BDSM, including empowerment, stress relief, emotional release, and self-exploration. BDSM can be a valuable tool for promoting personal growth, healing, and authenticity.

Encouragement for Continued Exploration and Growth in BDSM

As you continue your journey into BDSM, remember that exploration and growth are ongoing processes. Embrace curiosity, creativity, and self-discovery as you navigate new experiences and dynamics. Don't be afraid to push your boundaries, try new things, and communicate openly with your partner(s) about your desires, fears, and fantasies.

Cheryl Bach

Seek out supportive communities, resources, and mentors who can offer guidance, encouragement, and validation along the way. Remember that there's no one "right" way to do BDSM—every individual and relationship is unique, and it's okay to explore what works best for you and your partner(s).

Final Thoughts on the Potential of BDSM to Enhance Relationships and Personal Well-Being

BDSM has the potential to enrich relationships, deepen intimacy, and promote personal well-being in profound ways. By embracing trust, communication, and consent, individuals can create safe and empowering spaces for exploring desires, fantasies, and identities.

Through BDSM, individuals can cultivate greater self-awareness, resilience, and authenticity, leading to enhanced personal growth and fulfillment. Whether you're looking to spice up your sex life, strengthen your relationship, or embark on a journey of self-discovery, BDSM offers endless possibilities for exploration, connection, and transformation.

As you continue your exploration of BDSM, may you find joy, fulfillment, and empowerment in your experiences, and may you cultivate deeper connections and greater intimacy with yourself and your partner(s). Remember to prioritize safety, communication, and mutual respect in all your BDSM endeavors, and may your journey be as rewarding as it is exhilarating.

Thank you for embarking on this journey with us. May your future adventures in BDSM be filled with pleasure, passion, and personal growth.

Cheryl Bach